D1759785

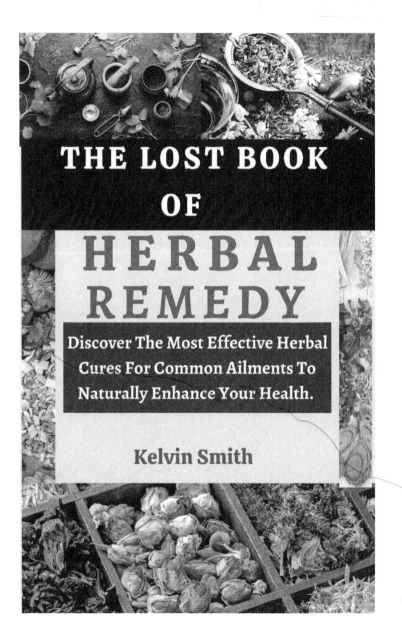

THE LOST BOOK

OF

HERBAL REMEDY

Discover The Most Effective Herbal Cures For Common Ailments To Naturally Enhance Your Health.

Kelvin Smith

THE LOST BOOK OF HERBAL REMEDY

Discover The Most Effective
Herbal Cures For Common
Ailments To Naturally Enhance
Your Health.

Kelvin Smith

All rights reserved. No part of this publication may be reproduced, distributed, or transmitted in any form or by any means, including photocopying, recording, or other electronic or mechanical methods, without the prior written permission of the publisher, except in the case of brief quotations embodied in critical reviews and certain other noncommercial uses permitted by copyright law.

Copyright © Kelvin Smith, 2022.

Table of Contents

Chapter 1

Getting to know the herbs

With so many herbs, treatments, and supplements on the market, all with varied and numerable advantages, it can sometimes be daunting to know where to start when it comes to building the proper regimen for your body and its requirements. So frequently patients expect herbalists to tell them "what they need" without asking themselves significant questions first. In this chapter I will shares what questions to ask yourself to identify the optimal herbal regimen for your body and mind.

Some of the most prevalent concerns that we encounters include digestive and gut health troubles, sleep and energy problems, brain health struggles when it comes to mood regulation, stress, and anxiety, overall wellbeing, and hormone imbalances. To start, it's crucial to recognize that there's no one size fits all herbal answer for everyone. It's crucial to look at your life and reflect on what support your body, brain, and lifestyle are demanding. Do you need treatment for a particular disease or a more preventive practice? Both are extremely vital, argues Robinett.

Next, you have to think about what is practical for you. What types of herbs will you stick to? How often? When? In what form? Everyone's daily routine is different, so check in with yourself to see what you can commit to since these remedies work most efficaciously when taken regularly, and there are so many options to choose from—a few big capsules, smaller capsules, teas, additions to your morning diet, changes to your nighttime routine, etc.

Herbs may be split into two groups. Accent herbs and plants lend character to recipes. Parsley, chives, and dill weed are a few of the accent herbs. They are gentler in taste and are commonly blended within the same dish. The character herbs; basil, marjoram, rosemary, bay leaves, thyme, sage, and tarragon lend dominating flavor to recipes.

Spiritual knowledge

Much traditional tribal information regarding plant treatment is based on intuition and dream knowledge. This metaphysical, or spiritual side of herbal treatment is possibly the toughest herbal information to understand for many. Like physiological knowing, it is a challenging sense to cultivate for individuals deeply entrenched in the rational and logical world.

Despite the Enlightenment being almost 200 years ago, there remains a dread in the West of subjective experience, leading to the contempt and scorn of both corporeal and spiritual knowledge. The term holistic is frequently reduced to merely mean 'alternative', while it truly refers to the full image, not only looking at a very tiny area of the whole.

As a herbalist, it's only when I access all three types of information, the scientific, the somatic sense, and the intuitive - that I can obtain a comprehensive and holistic understanding.

This is something we can all learn to accomplish, we simply need to combine the many aspects of ourselves, and our diverse methods of knowing. By learning to reconnect with ourselves and with plants, we're not just supporting our health, but our communities, and the planet herself.

Bodily knowing

A physiological understanding of herbs, the way plants taste, and the way that they feel on your tongue and in your body, comes from learning to pay attention profoundly. This type of physiological awareness is a talent to be taught and maintained, but it's available to everyone. The accumulation of this sort of information experienced and collected by many individuals over many centuries is what provides us with the body of knowledge that is traditional herbal literature and herbal wisdom.

Bodily knowledge may now be validated and supported by scientific information, but one without the other leads to an incomplete and superficial understanding of herbs and their connection to the body.

More so, a little heat unleashes the taste of herbs. Herbs are harsh, though, when cooked too much. Add accent herbs during the final five minutes of cooking time. Character herbs, like bay leaves, can endure lengthier cooking durations and normally are introduced at the beginning of the cooking process.

When purchasing fresh herbs, seek plants with an all-over green tint. Yellowing denotes elderly plants, whereas dark, wet spots are a symptom of damage.

To store fresh herbs for future use, rinse herbs under cold water, wipe dry, wrap in paper toweling, and chill in a plastic bag. To use, merely cut or take off leaves. Most refrigerated herbs will hold freshness for up to four days to a week.

Herbs may be frozen or dried for longer storage. To freeze fresh herbs, wash herbs, pat dry, and freeze in airtight bags or containers. Frozen herbs should be thawed only before usage. Fresh herbs may be dried for later use.

When experimenting with a new plant, pluck off a leaf and crush it, and let it warm in your palm. If it has a delicate scent you may add more. If it is harsh and smelly, use it sparingly. It is usually simpler to add more of a herb than to remove it.

Dried herbs are more concentrated. When cooking with dried herbs use one-third of the dried leaves to compensate for the fresh ones. One teaspoon of dried leaves is equivalent to one tablespoon of fresh. The fresh leaves are more pungent than the dry.

Chapter 2

herbal medicine preparation as a craft

Herbal Medicine making isn't only about finding the perfect herb, it's also about finding the right herbal preparation to utilize the herb effectively. From teas and tinctures to salves and soaps, finding the appropriate preparation may be challenging.

Chances are, even as an experienced home herbalist, there are quite a few herbal preparations you've never tried (and maybe never even heard of) (and maybe never even heard of).

Types of Herbal Preparations
A few varieties of herbal preparations.
Syrup, Comfrey Salve, Wort Tincture, and Pine Needle Tea.

Making herbal treatments is a little like baking in several respects. In the kitchen, the same few ingredients may produce everything from cakes to cookies and scones to sourdough. They're all presented in various ways and have their place in a meal.

When preparing medicinal herbs, you have a lot of possibilities in your home apothecary.

Most people are aware of herbal teas, but there are various ways that herbs are utilized medicinally, both topically and inwardly.

Some plants are better utilized topically, while others function best in beverages. Some contain water-soluble therapeutic qualities, while others require the alcohol from a tincture or to be infused into oil for extraction.

The therapeutic properties of several plants vary depending on the preparation.

The plant yarrow, for example, is used to halt bleeding and prevent infection when administered topically as a yarrow salve. When drunk as a tea, it's used internally to relieve symptoms of colds and flu.

The tea isn't going to assist your skinned knee any more than the salve is going to heal your cold. It's all about obtaining the correct herbal preparation.

Herbal Preparations of Yarrow in Four Different Herbal Preparations: Yarrow Tincture, Yarrow Herbal Beer, Yarrow Soap, and Yarrow Salve. All are used to cure various ailments, despite being manufactured with the same plant.

(Always check your doctor or a clinical herbalist before attempting any new herbal medicine, since there's always the risk of unforeseen effects, adverse responses, or combinations with other drugs. If you're picking wild plant material, make sure you're 100% certain in your identification and reference various sources for your ID. The following is based on my study and experience, but I don't pretend to have any credentials that would qualify me to advise you on your health. Please conduct your research and always check with numerous credible sources.)

Types Of HerbalPreparations
This basic list of herbal preparations includes the most frequent ways herbs are delivered. I'll go into each in detail soon.

Not every preparation is used with every plant, but here's a general overview of some of the alternatives available:

Fresh/Dried Herbs — Many herbs may be eaten straight out in the garden, or added as dried herbs to simmering cook pots in the kitchen.

Herbal Capsules

A handy method to consume dry herbs, herbal capsules allow for easy dosage.

Tea - Made by adding herbs to hot water, tea is one of the easiest herbal treatments.

Infusion - A strong tea brewed with either hot or cold water. They're frequently let to steep for several hours.

Decoction - A extremely powerful herbal tea created by decreasing the "tea" typically by as much as half its original volume to concentrate the therapeutic components.

Herbal Broth

Often created with medicinal mushrooms, or by putting herbs into conventional slow-cooked bone broths.

Herbal Steams - A little like a tea, in that boiling water is poured over herbs, but instead of drinking it, you inhale the vapor which is packed with the volatile oils of the herbs. This is very effective for respiratory disorders. This procedure is also occasionally utilized on other portions of the body, such as sore parts after delivery when they're still too wounded to apply a compress.

Poultice
Herbs are thoroughly chopped or crushed entirely before topical application.
Tincture - An alcohol extract of fresh or dried plant material. Most are single extraction tinctures created with only alcohol, but others employ a double extraction procedure that first extracts with alcohol and then water to draw out both the water and alcohol soluble elements.

Herbal Glycerite
Similar to a tincture, a glycerite employs vegetable glycerine instead of alcohol to generate a herbal extract. They're primarily employed by youngsters or persons avoiding alcohol.

Herbal Sprays ~
Usually comparable to a tincture, but packaged into a spray bottle for topical usage. Some of the most frequent are throat and mouth sprays, which are alcohol-based extracts placed into spray bottles for topical application on the mouth and throat. There are additional sprays used topically elsewhere for wound therapy and skin diseases as well.

Infused Oil
Dried herbs are infused into a carrier oil, which may be used internally or topically. It's most typically administered topically or used to manufacture herbal soaps, salves, or cosmetics.

Herbal Salve
Made by adding wax to a herbal infused oil to make a semi-solid herbal preparation that's simple to apply topically.

Herbs Soap
Often produced with herbal infused oil, a herbal soap is used topically to disinfect or cure skin diseases.

Bath Salts, Bath Bombs, and Sitz Baths — One broad set of herbal remedies that depend on sitting in a herbally infused bath. While bath bombs and salts normally indicate a full-body immersion in a tub, sitz baths are usually shallow water immersions for only one section of the body.

Infused Vinegar
Vinegar is used to retain plant material, and extract its therapeutic components comparable to a tincture.

Infused Honey
A little quantity of dried herbal material is put into honey and left to infuse. Usually 1 part herbs to 2-5 parts honey by volume.

Herbal Fermented Honey
When you add fresh herbs to honey (instead of dried), the herbs begin to ferment in the honey generating something that's halfway between mead and syrup. The fermentation makes certain herbs more bio-available and helps to preserve them at the same time.

Oxymel - A blend of herbs, vinegar, and honey that's consumed as a syrup. They're often a little more agreeable than plain herbal vinegar.

Herbal Syrups - Herbs are boiled with water and sugar or honey to form a delicious medicinal syrup.

Herbal Cough Drops & Lollypops -
In this recipe, herbs are boiled with sugar and honey to form hard candy that may be used as cough or throat drops.

Candied Herbs - Sometimes the herbs themselves are candied for preservation. Good examples include candied ginger and candied angelica, where the entire plant is soaked in sugar until it's preserved.

Jello & Gummies
These preparations are especially suitable for small children, who may not want to take their medication but may be encouraged to eat herbal jello for a sore throat or swallow elderberry gummies to aid with a cold. In certain situations, the natural gelatin that keeps them together actually has medicinal advantages too.

Electuary
A blend of honey and dried herbs, where enough dried herbal material is added such that the electuary may be made into herb and honey packets or tablets. It's essentially a botanical substance, only kept together with honey.

Compress
A cloth is soaked in a chilly herbal infusion and then applied topically.

Fomentation -

A cloth is soaked in a strong heat infusion and then applied topically. Similar to a compress, but administered heated so the heat is part of the therapy. They're most typically utilized for pain alleviation.

Succus - The newly produced juice of a plant, this preparation degrades fast. It was extensively used in the 1800s and prior when people visited the pharmacist to have fresh concoctions created on the spot. It's not often used anymore since it's not shelf-stable, so you won't find it at the drugstore. They may, however, be created simply at home.

Lacto-Fermented Herbs — Fresh green herbs may be Lacto-fermented, much like sauerkraut.

Herbal Wine, Mead, and Beer - Historically, herbal beers were one of the most prevalent herbal remedies. Back when everyone was brewing at home, instead of hops you would add other herbs which helped to flavor and preserve the beer but also were meant for therapeutic use. High-quality distilled alcohol for tinctures may have been costly, but any peasant could pick wild grapes and wild plants, combing them for homemade medicine.

Fresh and Dried Herbs
Many therapeutic herbs may be utilized immediately out of the garden, whether they're fresh or dried. There are various ways to utilize them without too much preparation.

For example, you may consume some herbs directly out of the garden to take care of small issues. Chewing on mint leaves generally decreases nausea, and occasionally simply smelling fresh rosemary leaves may have the same effect.

I used both of them to cure my morning sickness when I was pregnant with my first kid, and they worked great.

Fresh herbs deteriorate rapidly, so they'll need to be utilized in home cooking or straight out in the garden.

Keeping jars of dried herbs is one of the most adaptable methods to keep plants, and it's the base for many different herbal treatments.

They're utilized for practically every herbal product mentioned, from teas to tinctures and more. Those are extracts of course, which I'll address in a bit, but entire dried herbs may be used exactly as they are for herbal medicine as well.

Dried herbs may be used to make:
- Herbal Sleep Dream Pillows
- Mountain Rose Herbs
- Herbal Dryer Sachets

- The Rebooted Moms Natural Drawer Fresheners
- Wellness Mama's Immune Boosting Herbs

A collection of fresh and dried herbs that are proven to enhance the immune system.

Herbal Capsules
Dried herbs may be consumed orally in handmade herbal capsules.

Herbal capsules offer a few benefits:

You don't taste the herbs going down as you typically would with tea or tincture.
They may be carried anywhere, and you don't have to prepare boiling water like you would for tea.
Empty gelatin capsules are straightforward to fill with powdered herbs, however, the procedure is made easier using a capsule filling tray or small spatula developed for that purpose.

Herbal Teas

Most wannabe herbalists start with herbal teas since you can get readymade bags at the supermarket. I know I began by getting products like echinacea tea from the supermarket before I went into creating my own.

Herbal teas are one of the simplest herbal treatments. All you have to do is add the medicinal herbs to boiling water, allow it to soak, then drain and drink.

Try These Different Herbal Teas At Home.
- The Perfect Cup of Echinacea Tea
- Pine Needle Tea
- Sage Herbal Tea Recipe
- Marshmallow Root Tea
- Echinacea Tea
- Echinacea Tea
-

Infusion

An infusion is one of the most popular herbal preparations, and it's water-based, comparable to tea. Most infusions are created from the fragile parts of the plant, often termed the aerial components like the flowers, leaves, and stems.

It's easiest to think of an infusion as a powerful herbal tea produced with either cold or hot water that has been left to steep for several hours before using.

If you're new to medicinal herbs, infusions are one of the finest places to start; they're one of the simplest types of herbal preparations. It's excellent for novices.

Mountain Rose Herbs gives thorough instructions on how to produce both a hot and cold herbal infusion. This is a basic summary of the process:

Choose specific herbs to meet your therapeutic requirements. Grab a teapot and boil water. Then, pour the boiling water over the herbs and let them soak for at least an hour. If you wish to drink it hot, you may just reheat it. The longer that an infusion sets, the stronger it grows.

Some herbalists advocate using an overnight infusion with room temperature water since heat eliminates certain of the nutritional content in some kinds of herbs. Stinging nettle and red clover are often produced as room temperature infusions for that reason.

Here Are Some Examples OF Herbal Infusions.
- Stinging Nettle Infusion
- Dandelion Infusion
- Marshmallow Root Infusion
- Red Clover Infusion
- Red Clover Infusion
- Red Clover Infusion

Decoction

Decoctions are another water-based herbal preparation, but unlike infusions, they are often created with the bark, roots, seeds, and berries of the herbal plant. Some argue that decoctions are a powerful herbal tea, but it takes a lot more heat to create.

That's because when you produce a decoction, you're removing the active ingredients from the hard sections of the plant. That takes more time, and you have to compress the "tea" by as much as half its original volume to end up with the concentrated ingredients.

Take anywhere between a teaspoon and a tablespoon of herbal stuff (per cup of water) and put it in a pot. Make sure the herb is powdered, split, or crushed into little bits. It shouldn't be huge portions.
Add a cup of water, and bring it to a boil. Then, decrease the heat and let it simmer for 15 minutes.

After it's cooked, drain the decoction through a fine-mesh sieve or cheesecloth. It should be consumed when still hot.

These are Different Herbal Decoctions:
Echinacea Decoction
Spring Cleansing Decoction

Herbal Broth
Similar to decoctions, herbal broths are gently cooked extracts. They may be integrated into cooking, or just put into a cup and drunk.

Simply adding medicinal herbs to a slow-simmered homemade bone broth will work, and enables you to utilize your food as medicine. In such a situation, you need to be cautious to choose herbs with a pleasing taste.

The most popular herbal broth is a medicinal mushroom soup, generally produced with exceedingly hard-to-extract species such as Chaga, Reishi, and Turkey Tail Mushrooms.

Herbal Steams
Usually utilized to extract volatile chemicals, herbal steams are commonly used for respiratory ailments.

Boiling water is poured over fragrant plants and then the ensuing vapor is softly breathed.

My favorite herbal steam is created with thyme, which works great for cleaning the sinuses.

Beyond thyme, there are dozens of plants typically used in herbal steams, including peppermint, lavender, eucalyptus, cinnamon, basil, chamomile, and pine needles.

Poultices

Poultices are created from fresh or dried herbs that are soaked and coarsely crushed or pulverized before being used as a topical treatment. One of the most frequent poultices is created using the plantain herb to be administered for insect bites and stings.

Poultices also aid with burns, rashes, strains, sprains, inflammation, and many other skin ailments.

There are numerous sorts of poultices that you may produce.

Astringent poultices are used to assist pull out foreign items, such as a splinter or glass piece. They also assist to pull out pus or debris from wounds by boosting the circulation of the skin.

Heating poultices soothe muscles and improve circulation and warmth to an area. These are most typically administered to bruises, strains, sprains, and other muscular disorders. However, you must be cautious while using a hot poultice since it might cause skin irritation or burning.

Vulnerary poultices are created using demulcent herbs because of their calming properties. They're most typically utilized for inflammation, rashes, or abrasions.
When you construct a poultice, you'll apply it directly on the surface of your skin, often up to an inch thick, and hold it in place using gauze or muslin wrapped around the region. Some people don't like poultices because they take longer to work and are messier than salves or ointments, but a poultice is a terrific alternative for utilizing fresh herbs in the field.

Here's how you prepare a poultice.

Decide whether you want to use fresh or dried herbs and how much of the herbs you need to use is dependent on the size of the area you want to cover. If you're using fresh herbs, you'll need to cut them up into little bits. A mortar and pestle assist to grind the herbs and get the juices flowing.

Spread the herbs over the skin region and cover the area with gauze or muslin to retain your poultice in place. If you use dry herbs, you'll need to mix them with a touch of boiling water to help make a paste.

Tincture
Tinctures are highly concentrated herbal medicines created by extracting the active components of the medicinal plant with a combination of alcohol and water. Typically, tinctures are the most popular preparation utilized by naturopaths and herbalists since they're highly effective.

Most are single extraction tinctures created using simply alcohol. Still, some utilize a twofold extraction procedure that first extracts with alcohol and then water to draw out both the water and alcohol soluble elements. A reishi mushroom tincture is an example of a double extraction tincture.

If you're producing tinctures at home, I advise beginning with a single extraction. However, tinctures take time to create, so you have to have patience. Remember, they are also considerably stronger than infusions or decoctions, so they need to be taken in much lower dosages.

Here's how to produce a tincture at home.

Start by placing finely chopped medicinal herbs into a glass container. For tinctures, any parts of the plant may be utilized. Then, pour alcohol over the plant stuff and seal up the container. Keep this in the container for four to six weeks, stirring the jar frequently.

After the time limit is up, strain the tincture through a fine-mesh strainer and put it back into a clean glass jar. Tinctures should be kept in a dark cabinet for the best-prolonged shelf life.

Here are some Different Herbal Tinctures:
- Yarrow Tincture
- Elderberry Tincture
- Black Walnut Tincture
- Burdock Tincture
- Dandelion Tincture
- Chickweed Tincture

Reishi Mushroom Tincture infusing in mason jars, as the first phase (alcohol extraction) of a double extraction tincture.

Herbal Glycerites
Typically termed glycerin-based extractions, glycerites are swiftly becoming a popular choice for parents who don't want to use alcohol-based tinctures for their children. Using glycerin enables you to generate a sweeter, more appealing extract, but they aren't as strong as alcohol-based tinctures.

Something you should remember before getting started is that herbal glycerites have a significantly shorter shelf life, and they are best kept in the refrigerator.

You need to have food-grade vegetable glycerin, a clear, odorless liquid that originates from vegetable oils.

When preparing glycerites, you want to use fresh herbs since glycerin is excellent at keeping fresh plant fluids, but if you only have dried herbs, that work as well.

Here's how to create a herbal glycerite at home.

Start with a clean glass jar and add your chopped fresh herbs, filling the container as much as possible. If you use dried herbs, don't fill the jar since dry materials expand more. Then, add enough glycerin to thoroughly cover the plant material to within one inch of the top.

Use a spoon to probe at the plant material and expel any air bubbles. Then, cover the jar with the lid and place it in a dark spot at room temperature. It takes between four to six weeks for glycerites to be finished, and make sure you shake the container once or twice every day.

After the infusing is done, strain the glycerite through a fine-mesh sieve or a few layers of cheesecloth. Then, put it back in a labeled, clean jar.

Here Are a Few Glycerite Recipes to Try.
- Peach Flower Glycerite
- Violet Flower Glycerite
- Honeysuckle Glycerite
- Homemade Glycerite for a Fever
- Making Chamomile Glycerite

Herbal Sprays
A tincture in a spray bottle, herbal sprays are a practical method to administer herbal

treatments topically. That can imply "topically" inside your mouth and throat for a herbal sore throat spray, or topically to cuts and wounds as with a yarrow spray.

Generally, herbal sprays are alcohol-based extracts so that they're kept shelf-stable. The additional alcohol also helps to operate as a topical disinfectant, serving to both preserve the herbs and assist them to heal symptoms on the skin.

Sometimes, like with herbal throat sprays, raw honey will be used to increase taste and as an extra antimicrobial.

Beyond direct topical usage, herbal sprays are sometimes employed as insect repellants and aromatherapy sprays. We also produce a tea tree deodorant spray that's effective, just combining witch hazel and a few drops of tea tree oil.

Anything herbal in a spray bottle qualifies as a herbal spray.

Infused Oil

For some of the most versatile herbal preparations, herbal-infused oils are the initial step to preparing all kinds of other herbal medicines.

You may use them directly on the skin or use them to produce herbal salves, herbal soaps, and ointments. Infused oils are wonderful for nourishing dry skin, and relieving irritated skin, inflammation, or muscular ache.

Infused oils are prepared by infusing dry herbs into a carrier oil. These may be used orally or topically; some choose to use infused oils for recipes since they improve the taste of foods.

Making herbal infused oils is one of the simplest kinds of herbal preparations, therefore it's excellent for beginners. It starts by taking a carrier oil and your favorite dried medicinal herb. However, it takes time to manufacture herbal-infused oils, so you need some patience.

Start by filling your glass jar with the therapeutic plant or herbs of your choice. Fill the jar, allowing at least an inch of room at the top. Don't worry; the oil has plenty of room to fill up. Now, pour in the oil that you picked, leaving room at the top between the lid and oil.

Store this in a cold, dark spot, such as your kitchen cupboard, and remember to shake it periodically. After four to six weeks, rinse off the dried herbs and store your infused oils.

Herbal Salve
Once you have an infused herbal oil, you blend it with beeswax to form a herbal salve. Herbal salves are thicker than ointments, but it helps them remain on the skin longer.

They are manufactured by adding wax to a herbal infused oil to make a semi-solid herbal treatment that's simple to apply topically. Herbal salves are a simple but efficient method to employ herbs. It's simple to slip a jar of salve in your handbag or diaper bag, and because they're semi-solid, they aren't as messy.

You may manufacture herbal salves using a single herb or herbal mixes. You can come up with any combination you desire for whatever you need.

Herbal Soap
If you have herbal infused oil, you may utilize it to produce herbal soaps that can be used topically to cure skin issues, disinfect wounds, and other beneficial purposes. You may also prepare herbal soaps utilizing herbal teas, infusions, tinctures, fresh or dried herbs, and decoctions.

Learning how to create herbal soap is a terrific way to use up stuff in your medical herbal cabinet. I occasionally make soap with my handmade witch hazel extract; you can use it to create this yarrow and witch hazel herbal soap.

People are generally too scared about starting into manufacturing soap at home. Working with lye may be challenging, but with the correct safety measures, it can be immensely gratifying.

Here Are Some Different Herbal Soap Recipes to Try:
- Creamy Chickweed Soap
- Honey & Dandelion Soap Recipe
- Herbal Soap with Rosemary and Peppermint
- Chamomile Lavender and Eucalyptus Soap
- Herbal Gardeners Soap with Spring Weeds

- Gardeners Soap with Spring Weeds from Easy Melt and Pour Soaps
- Gardeners Soap with Spring Weeds (Photo Credit Jan Berry)

Bath Salts, Bath Bombs & Sitz Baths
The bath is an easy method to apply herbs topically, and the warm water is frequently wonderfully calming. Add in a fizzy herbal bath bomb or some scented bath salts and you've converted a peaceful soak into a herbal treatment session.

Sitz baths are similar, but they're more focused. Usually, a sitz bath is used to submerge painful portions to treat postpartum difficulties or hemorrhoids, and only one part of the body is immersed in water.

Infused Vinegar Or Vinegar Extractions
Vinegar-based herbal treatments are another popular alternative since they bring out more of the nutrients and mineral profiles in the plants. These have a lengthy

shelf life, comparable to tinctures prepared in alcohol, so you may expect to have them around for a long time.

Herbal vinegar is a fantastic alternative if you have upper respiratory difficulties, such as a sore throat or congestion. You may use infused vinegar-like tinctures or add them to infusions and decoctions after being created separately.

The most popular method to utilize infused vinegar is while cooking. They taste fantastic on vegetables and salads but don't shy away from using them to heal diseases. A dear friend of mine claims that her vinegar-based extractions halted her itchy scalp condition in its tracks!

One of the nicest things about producing herbal forms of vinegar is that you can use whatever sort of vinegar you have, whether it's apple cider vinegar, white vinegar, rice vinegar, or any other variety. That's why it's such a popular option for gourmet meals; the mix of tastes is virtually unlimited.

Here's how to produce herbal vinegar.

Start with a big quart jar and add one cup of dry herbs; use one kind of herb or a mix of your favorites. Feel free to experiment! Then, add two glasses of the vinegar you picked. Cover the jar with the lid, but maintain a layer of waxed paper beneath if using a metal cover since the vinegar causes the metal to rust.

Vinegar-based extractions take up to one month to infuse. Make careful to shake the jar periodically and start tasting after one week.

After you have the taste wanted, take a glass jar or container to keep your freshly completed herbal vinegar. These bottles need to be kept in a cold, dark area.

Here Are Some Infused Herbal Vinegar:
Lavender-Rosemary Herbal Vinegar
Elderberry-Infused Herbal Vinegar
Infused Dandelion Vinegar
Bee Balm Vinegar
Nasturtium Infused Vinegar

Infused Honey
Without a doubt, infused honey is perhaps the sweetest herbal preparation choice, and it's highly effective. Infused honey helps to cure sore throats, remove infections, and act on a damaged immune system.

Honey itself is useful when you have a sickness. It's a natural emollient, demulcent, and has nutritional advantages. The demulcent characteristics make it good for calming coughs and soothing dry, sore throats. If you're having problems swallowing because your throat aches, honey is the way to go.

When preparing an infused honey, you add a small number of herbs to the honey and let them infuse. It's normally suggested to use a ratio of one part herbs to two to five parts honey depending on the amount you have.

Be sure to use dried herbs for infusions, as the moisture in fresh herbs will cause the honey to ferment. (We'll explore fermented honey preparations next...)

Fermented Honey
While dried herbs create herbal infused honey, the moisture in fresh herbs may be utilized to make herbal fermented honey.

Honey already includes natural yeast, but it doesn't ferment because the sugar content is too high. Add a lot of water and you may easily produce mead (honey wine) at home.

Add just a touch of moisture in the form of herbs or berries, and you'll get gently fermented herbal honey instead.

Some herbs are more bio-available once they've been fermented. Turmeric is a wonderful example, and fermented turmeric is a potent anti-inflammatory. Adding fresh turmeric to honey is one technique to ferment this plant.

Here are a couple more nice possibilities for herbal fermented honey:

Oxymel
An oxymel is a blend of herbs, vinegar, and honey that you consume like a syrup. It's most typically used as a herbal preparation to conceal the taste of strong aromatic herbs, such as garlic and pepper.

Fire cider is arguably the best-known oxymel, although there are numerous more.

Taking an oxymel is far more enjoyable than a straight-infused herbal vinegar.

Most oxymel remedies are created using a mix of apple cider vinegar and raw honey. These are two commonplace kitchen ingredients, and most herbalists use this to settle an unpleasant cough, relieve a sore throat, and improve your weakening immune system.

An oxymel isn't as widespread as other herbal remedies these days, but historically, it was an immensely popular herbal cure. As more individuals begin to know the medicinal potential of both raw cider vinegar and raw honey, homemade oxymels are coming back into favor among the herbal community.

Herbal Syrups
Herbal syrups are an old-fashioned sort of herbal concoction often created to aid with sore throats, coughs, colds, and other mucus-related upper respiratory disorders.

Syrups are often a sweeter herbal treatment, great for youngsters to ingest.

Instead of purchasing syrups from the supermarket (that cost an arm and a leg), you may prepare your herbal syrups based on what diseases your family has.

These are some Different Herbal Syrups you can make.
- Homemade Elderberry Syrup
- Wild Cherry Bark Syrup
- Pine Needle Cough Syrup
- Honey Thyme Cough Syrup
- Homemade Elderberry Syrup
- Homemade Elderberry Syrup
-

Herbal Cough Drops & Lollypops
Cook a herbal syrup down a little more, and you'll have hard candy for herbal cough drops or lollypops.

Hard cough drops are simpler to travel than syrups, and they dissolve slowly in your mouth so they keep a cough (or sore throat) at bay longer.

Herbal lollipops are very much the same thing, but particularly tempting to youngsters.

Horehound Cough Drops
Elderberry Lolly Pops
Homemade elderberry lollipops prepared with elderberry syrup

Electuary
Almost like infused honey, an electuary is powdered herbs blended with honey till it forms a paste. The herbal honey paste may then be eaten off a spoon, poured into hot water to produce something like tea, or simply wrapped in a little more herb powder to form mini electuary "pills."
Honey has all sorts of helpful, therapeutic characteristics on its own, so when you mix

it with a variety of powdered herbs, it's a strong, shelf-stable herbal concoction.

Taking an electuary is simple because it tastes so wonderful, so it's excellent for youngsters. You also may warm it up and combine it with a little water or add it to a cup of tea. Some additionally utilize an electuary to mold into honey packets or pills; it's a new technique to practice encapsulation.

Here's how to create an electuary at home.

Start with powdered herbs and put them into a bowl. Slowly pour the honey into the basin and whisk. Keep stirring and adding honey until you get a thick paste. If you prefer a thinner product, feel free to add extra honey.
Once you get the consistency that you desire, keep it in a clean jar and seal firmly. It's advised to store in your fridge for up to 12 months, but because the herbs are

combined with honey, I assume the shelf-life is considerably longer than that.

Fomentation And Compresses

Sometimes termed a compress, a fomentation employs infusions or decoctions to make a topical treatment. Compresses and fomentations are commonly used similarly, but the difference is temperature. Compresses are normally made cold whereas fomentations are produced hot.

The temperature utilized matters dependent on why you need a fomentation. Hot fomentations release tight muscles and circulate circulation to the skin, minimizing interior congestion and healing aching muscles. Cold fomentations constrict blood vessels, therefore this is good for acute burns, bruising, and inflammation.

No matter what form of fomentation you apply, they are utilized for skin concerns.

They're wonderful for rashes, eczema, and other disorders.

Here are basic methods for producing herbal fomentations.

Start with three to four teaspoons of medicinal herbs per one cup of water. Let this soak for up to 30 minutes, and then filter the herbs out of the liquid using a cheesecloth. Feel free to add a few drops of tincture per cup as well.

Take a clean piece of cloth and immerse it into the heated infusion, wringing away the excess liquid. Apply this to the troubled region; you'll instantly feel pleasant alleviation. When it cools, dip it into the infusion again and reapply.

If you wish to apply a cold compress rather than a heated fomentation, wait for the infusion or decoction to cool before dipping the cloth and utilizing it.

Here Are examples of Compresses And Fomentation.

Bone Healing Comfrey Compress
Chamomile Compress for Hay Fever Relief
Homemade Compress for Pain, Fever, and Cramps
Mastitis Compress with Mullein

Succus

One of the least frequent herbal preparations is termed succus, the freshly produced juice of a plant or its fruit. Most manufacturers in the herbal sector do not supply it since the juice has to be fresh. Instead, home herbalists more typically utilize Succi.

While tinctures are regarded as a much stronger herbal preparation, a succus is a helpful choice for utilizing an excess of therapeutic plants.

Ideally, you'll have a juicer or something to utilize to generate your succus. All you have to do is add the herbs, along with fruits and vegetables into your juicer, but if you don't have a juicer, producing a succus is still doable. You'll have to mix the ingredients and filter them through a cheesecloth.

The ideal method to consume a herbal succus is to drink it as a fresh juice, but it also may be saved to be employed later. Traditionally, herbalists used 25% alcohol by volume to preserve the fresh juice, while some add a succus to tinctures to boost the strength.

Other times, herbalists make succi for exterior purposes. For example, you can freeze them until you need them. A nice example of this is frozen jewelweed cubes for bug bites.

Making a succus isn't that popular anymore, but if you have vast quantities of herbs that you have no clue how to utilize, this is an excellent solution. Also, it's good when you have a lot of wild plants that you foraged. Some of the greatest plants for a succus are chickweed, calendula, plantain, dandelions, elderberries, and ginger.

Lacto fermented Herbs
Similar to homemade sauerkraut, fresh herbs may be Lacto-fermented.

Fermenting herbs will preserve them, similar to the way fermentation preserves vegetables, but it also makes certain herbs more bioavailable.

This issue is a little delicate, since certain plants may turn harmful when fermented. Good examples of that include melilot (or sweet clover), which becomes a blood thinner when fermented. Cherry bark, similarly turns poisonous when fermented, although it's a classic herbal cough treatment otherwise.

If you want to ferment herbs, make sure you know the influence of fermentation on the specific plant in question.

Herbal Wine , Mead , And Beer
Long ago beer, wine, and mead were more than simply a means to spend a Friday night with friends.

Herbs were fermented into alcoholic drinks to retain their therapeutic virtues. This was back when just about everyone produced beer at home to sanitize water and putting in medicinal plants helped to heal common diseases at the same time.

These days, hops are omnipresent in beer, but traditionally they weren't used all that much. Instead, numerous wild plants were employed to flavor and preserve the beer while also imparting therapeutic benefits.

Today this is known as "Gruit" or herbal beer.

The same was true of wine and mead, and frequently there was no differentiation between the three forms of alcohol. Our predecessors would toss in malted grains, crushed fruits, and honey all together to produce mixed drinks, and these mish-mash brews are by far the most prevalent in the archeological record.

These days we're frequently purists when it comes to beer vs. wine vs. mead, but back in the day, they didn't make such a difference. The book Ancient Brews: Rediscovered and Recreated includes some intriguing archeological investigations (and recipes) that cover ancient brews in depth.

We're major brewing geeks, and I spend a lot of time reading about this topic. If you're interested in herbal brewing, I'd also recommend:

Any Other Herbal Preparations ?

I've attempted to cover every sort of popular (and not so common) herbal preparation accessible, but I'm constantly astonished to discover new approaches.

Disclaimer On Homemade Herbal Remedies

I've been harvesting natural medicines and treating my family with herbal cures for the last 15 years, but I'm self-taught. Be aware that I am not a clinical herbalist, and everything is based on my study and personal experience utilizing medicinal herbs. I do not pretend to have the expertise that'd qualify me to counsel you on your health, and I'm merely presenting this as a reference to inspire a greater interest in medicinal plants.

Please use this as a jumping-off point, but always conduct your research and verify everything you read with numerous sources.

It's always possible to have a bad response to any medicinal plant, and lots of individuals are sensitive to even benign herbs like chamomile. Always check your doctor or a professional herbalist before attempting any new medicinal plant. Often, they might have unanticipated responses in conjunction with other herbs and vitamins, and many herbs have side effects even when they are helpful for their original purpose.

Chapter 3

9-leading edge herbs

Today, we live in a period where produced drugs and prescriptions rule, but do they have to be the sole path to healing?

Even with all of these sophisticated alternatives at our fingertips, many individuals find themselves coming back to the medical plants that began it all: Herbal medicines that have the power to cure and promote physical and mental well-being.

In fact, at the beginning of the 21st century, 11 percent of trusted sources of the 252 medications classified "basic and essential" by the World Health Organization were "exclusively of flowering plant origin." Drugs like codeine, quinine, and morphine all include plant-derived components.

While these manmade pharmaceuticals have become crucial in our lives, it might be pleasant to know that the power of nature is on our side, and these herbal options are there to supplement our health practices.

But the amount of influence they possess is still being investigated. These alternatives aren't cure-alls, and they aren't flawless. Many contain the same dangers and negative effects as industrial drugs. Many of them are offered unsubstantiated promises.

However, many plants and drinks provide safe subtle methods to boost your health. Pay attention to what the data indicates about each herb's efficacy as well as any interactions or safety risks. Avoid using herbs for babies and children and for individuals who are pregnant and nursing. Most herbs haven't been studied for safety for individuals who are susceptible, and using herbs isn't worth the risk.

With this cautionary story in mind, picking the correct plant might seem challenging to someone who just wants to feel better without using the medicine. That's why, with my experiment, I focus on looking into

the most effective and therapeutic herbs –
which have good scientific evidence to back
their safe usage.

Making judgments concerning herbs
combined with more conventional
therapeutic techniques is something you
and your healthcare practitioner may handle
together.

At times, I observe, consuming the plants
might be even less dangerous than taking
concentrated, produced supplements since
there's a greater possibility of contamination
of the substance with the production
procedures. It's a fantastic way to feel their
benefits and the delight of cultivating them
yourself. Herbs may also be a means to
provide a required nutrient.

However, both plants and supplements,
which aren't controlled by the Food and
Drug Administration for safety or quality,
might have dubious doses and can have a

danger of contamination. Keep this in mind while purchasing supplements from the shelves.

If you'd like to add some medicinal plants to your health routine, research sorts through the latest findings and gives a scoring system for our selection.

These plants have the most numerous high-quality research and are the safest alternatives among herbal treatments.

We hope this guide will work as a beginning point for individuals who seek to incorporate herbal treatments into their life and come prepared with information. As always, talk with your doctor before beginning any new health therapy.

Gingko

As one of the oldest tree species, ginkgo is also one of the oldest homeopathic plants and a significant herb in Chinese medicine. The leaves are used to manufacture capsules, pills, and extracts, and when dried, may be eaten as tea.

It's arguably best-known for its potential to promote brain health. Studies show that ginkgo can help individuals with mild to moderate dementia Trusted Source, and may decrease memory decline in dementia and Alzheimer's disease.

Recent research is looking at a component that might aid diabetes, and there continue to be additional studies, including an animal study that shows it can improve bone mending.

The ginkgo tree is considered a living fossil, having remains dating from 270 million years ago. These trees may live up to 3,000 years.

Gingko might be good for:

- Dementia
- Alzheimer's disease
- eye health
- inflammation
- diabetes
- bone healing
- anxiety
- depression

Things to put under consideration

- Long-term usage may raise the probability of thyroid and liver cancer, which has been demonstrated in rats.
- It's known to be taxing on the liver, therefore liver enzymes may need to be checked.
- It may interact with blood thinners.
- Gingko seeds are toxic if swallowed.
- Side effects might include headache, upset stomach, dizziness, and allergic response.
- Gingko usage has to be addressed with your doctor because of various medication interactions.

Turmeric

With its striking orange color, it's tough to miss a bottle of turmeric lying on a spice rack. Originating in India, turmeric is considered to have anticancer effects and may prevent DNA abnormalities.

As an anti-inflammatory, it may be taken as a supplement and it's been used topically for patients with arthritis who seek to ease suffering. It's utilized internationally as a culinary ingredient, which makes it a wonderful, antioxidant-richTrusted Source addition to many cuisines.

According to the current study, turmeric is also showing promise as a therapy for several dermatologic illnesses and joint arthritisTrusted Source.

Turmeric has been used as a medicinal herb for 4,000 years. It's a tentpole of an Indian alternative medicine technique called Ayurveda.

Turmeric might be good for:
- pain caused by inflammatory disorders, such arthritis
- preventing cancer
- stopping DNA abnormalities
- various skin disorders

Things to put under consideration
- When taken as a supplement, individuals tend to take too much, therefore it might be difficult to trust the quantity and quality. Safety rises when taken as a herb in cooking or tea.
- Long-term usage might cause gastric troubles.
- Turmeric has limited bioavailability. Consuming with pepper may help your body absorb more of its advantages.

Rating

The vivid yellow evening primrose flower generates oil that's supposed to relieve the symptoms of PMS and skin disorders like dermatitis.

Some that are accessible on this oil seem to be all over the map, however, some studies are stronger than others. For example, several research has revealed that evening primrose oil has anti-inflammatory benefits. It's been found to aid with illnesses such as atopic dermatitis and diabetic neuropathyTrusted Source. It may also aid

with other health conditions, such as breast discomfort.

A recent study suggests increasing the quality of life for individuals with multiple sclerosisTrusted Source, altering hormones and insulin sensitivity in those suffering from the polycystic ovarian syndrome, and applying it topically to relieve moderate dermatitis.

According to these findings, evening primrose oil could well be the Swiss Army knife of the therapeutic plant world. The drawback is that it may interfere with numerous drugs. More research is coming, and the applications seem exciting.

Evening primrose blooms are often called moonflowers because they bloom as the sun starts to set. People frequently remark they smell like lemons.

Evening primrose oil might be effective for:
- minor skin conditions
- breast pain
- menopause
- inflammation
- diabetic neuropathy

- multiple sclerosis
- PCOS
- blood pressure

Things to put under consideration
- interacts with certain blood-clotting medications
- safety during pregnancy is uncertain
- may interfere with drug absorption during HIV treatment
- Interacts with lithium for bipolar disorder
- long-term usage may not be safe

Flax seed

Flax seed, also available as an oil, is one of the safest alternatives among plant-based nutritional supplements. Harvested for thousands of years, nowadays flax seed is renowned for its antioxidant activity and anti-inflammatory effects.

Although more research has to be done with human participants, one study shows that flax seeds may help prevent colon cancer.

Another study trusted by sources claims that flaxseed can lower blood pressure. When ingested, it may potentially assist in lowering obesity. Many people add flax seed and flaxseed powder to oatmeal and smoothies, and it's also available in the form of pills, oil (which may be put into capsules), and flour.

The best method to incorporate flax seed is via your diet. Sprinkle ground seeds over cereal or salad, simmer in hot cereal, stew, handmade slices of bread, or smoothies. Add flaxseed oil to salad dressing.

Flax seeds are one of a handful of plant-based sources of omega-3 fatty acids.

Other sources include chia seeds, walnuts, and soybeans.

Flax seed might be good for :
- decreasing obesity
- regulating blood pressure
- avoiding colon cancer
- inflammation
- hot flushes

Things to put under consideration
Flax seeds may alter estrogen production in women, particularly if they have a history of cancer or are pregnant.
Don't consume raw or unripe flax seeds, since they might be poisonous.

Tea tree oil

The tea tree, which is native to Australia, produces an oil that's long been regarded to be good for skin ailments, including moderate acne, athlete's foot, tiny wounds, dandruff, insect bites, and other inflammatory skin disorders.

There has to be a greater investigation into acne and scalp usage, but for now, there's a degree of research into the antibacterial properties of tea tree oil on wounds and topical infections.

One recent research indicated that tea tree oil inhibited the development of acne-causing bacteria. It's often utilized as a highly concentrated essential oil.

Wilson says that tea tree oil, like other essential oils, should be diluted in a carrier oil. She notes that it typically already comes diluted in several skin care products and lotions.

Tea tree oil is obtained from the leaves of a tree that's native to Queensland and New South Wales, Australia.

Tea tree oil might be good for:
- acne
- athlete's foot
- cuts
- dandruff
- insect bites

Things to put under consideration
- Tea tree oil is toxic if consumed orally.
- Your skin might develop an allergic response.
- It may alter hormones.
- Long-term usage isn't encouraged.

Echinacea

Echinacea is a lot more than the gorgeous, purple coneflowers you see dotting gardens. These blossoms have been utilized for generations as medicine in the form of teas, juice, and extracts. Today, they may be taken as powders or supplements.

The best-known application of echinacea is to lessen symptoms of the common coldTrusted Source, but further research is required to validate this effect and to understand how echinacea improves immunity when a virus is present.

Generally, except for a few minor adverse effects, echinacea is quite harmless. Even if it requires additional testing, you may always opt to utilize it if you're expecting to see your cold symptoms disappear more rapidly.

Some of the first humans to employ echinacea as a therapeutic plant were Native Americans. The earliest archaeological evidence goes back to the 18th century.

Echinacea might be good for:
- colds
- immunity
- bronchitis
- upper respiratory infections

Things to put under consideration

- It may be harsh on the digestive system and upset the stomach.
- Allergic responses are possible.

Grape Seed extract

For years, grape seed extract, which is accessible as liquid, pills, or capsules, has been well-established and recognized for its antioxidant activities. It offers strong health advantages, including decreasing LDL (bad) cholesterol and improving signs of impaired circulation in the leg veins.

StudiesTrusted Source is demonstrating that frequent ingestion of grapeseed extract has anticancer benefits and tends to inhibit cancer cell proliferation.

Grapeseed extract includes the same antioxidants found in wine.

Grapeseed extract might be good for:
- cancer

- lowering LDL (bad) cholesterol
- leg vein circulation
- edema
- blood pressure

Things to put under consideration
- Proceed with care if you use blood thinners or blood pressure drugs, or if you're preparing to go in for surgery.
- It may limit iron absorption.

Lavender

If you feel anxiety, chances are that someone along the line has advised that you use lavender essential oil, and for good reason. This aromatic, purple flower has a fairly strong standing among studies, which have mainly focused on its anti-anxiety capacities.

It's proven to be soothing in a study conducted among dental patients, while another study confirmed that lavender can directly impact mood and cognitive performance. It's also been commended for its sedative properties to help people get much-needed sleep.

Recently, it's been shown that lavender contains anti-inflammatory effects as well. It's best effective diluted and applied on the skin or used in aromatherapy, and it has few adverse effects.

Lavender was initially introduced to Provence, France, by the Romans 2,000 years ago.

Lavender might be good for:
- anxiety
- stress
- blood pressure
- migraine

Things to consider
- It may cause skin inflammation.
- It's toxic if taken orally.

- It may alter hormones when administered undiluted.

Chamomile

With blooms that resemble miniature daisies, chamomile is another medicinal plant that's claimed to offer anti-anxiety qualities. Most people know it since it's a popular tea taste (one review trusted Source indicates that over 1 million cups per day are eaten throughout the globe), but it may also be absorbed via liquids, capsules, or tablets.

The soothing properties of chamomile have been repeatedly examined, including a 2009 study trusted Source that indicates chamomile is preferable to using a placebo while treating generalized anxiety disorder. One recent research verified it's safe for long-term usage, while another recent study trusted Source went beyond its use for anxiety and found that it also has promise in anticancer therapies.

There are two forms of chamomile: German chamomile, an annual that flourishes in the Midwest, and Roman chamomile, a perennial that attracts pollinators and smells like apples.

Chamomile might be good for:
- anxiety
- stress
- insomnia
- cancer

Things to put under consideration
- It may induce allergic responses. There've been reports of anaphylaxis.
- It may interact with blood thinners.

Chapter 4

Assembling your first aid kit and domestic herb cabinet

Despite our best endeavors to live a healthy and toxin-free life, there are occasions when disease or injury strikes. In some of these circumstances (like trauma), traditional medical therapy is necessary, and I'm certainly thankful that medical treatment is accessible if needed.

But what about the instances when the disease or injury is not life-threatening, but rather inconvenient or limiting?

The following is a list of everything you'll find in my "medicine" cupboard and natural first aid kit. It is a blend of cures I've tried myself, ones advised by a naturopathic doctor, and ones that I hope to never use!

Remedies & Herbs in My Natural First Aid Kit.
Before we start, bear in mind that I didn't set up this list overnight! It took many years of study and trial and error to uncover the medicines I use and trust the most.

Activated Charcoal:
For acute usage in food poisoning, intestinal sickness, vomiting, diarrhea, intake of poisons, etc. Also, have the local poison control number on hand in case a kid ingests a dangerous chemical and promptly send a child to the hospital if he/she has ingested a battery or magnet!

Arnica:
Topical cream used for muscular discomfort or damage, bruising, or any form of trauma. We've discovered that it substantially improved healing time or bruising and tight muscles when taken topically shortly after an incident. Not for internal usage or use on open wounds.

Homeopathics :
Along with arnica (above), I have a supply of Genexa homeopathic pills on hand for aiding kids with sleep, cold relief, and even anxiety.

Cayenne Powder:

Though this is an excellent complement to many dishes, it's even better to keep in a medical cabinet. I have a couple of cayenne pills in my bag as well.

Topically, cayenne pepper helps stop bleeding fast. I've heard reports of it being taken internally during heart attacks to enhance blood flow and assist remove the obstruction, but happily, I've never had to try this one. It is also a great medicine to take internally during sickness as it is proven to boost blood flow and expedite healing (however I do not offer it to youngsters) (although I do not give it to children).

Chamomile:

I use it to prepare a calming tincture that helps calm youngsters whether they are unwell or simply have difficulties sleeping. The medication also works great on teething gums. The dried flowers may also be formed into a poultice with some gauze and applied on an eye for 15 minutes every hour to help alleviate pink eye (typically works in a couple of hours) (usually works in a couple of hours). Brewed as a tea, chamomile is a pleasant drink at night and the tea may be chilled and put on the stomach of colicky newborns to help comfort them. I occasionally add some brewed chamomile tea to the kid's bath since it is beneficial for the skin and encourages calm. I have the tincture in my handbag at all times.

Comfrey:

An external herb that aids healing from injuries and fractured bones. A poultice composed of plantain and comfrey that is applied to a wound may considerably decrease the healing period and help prevent and cure the infection. I create a homemade "Neosporin" using this and other herbs and use it for insect bites, scratches, bruises, and poison ivy. It is recommended to have the dried herb on hand for poultices and homemade salves.

Eucalyptus Herb and Essential Oils:
I have them in my natural first aid bag for respiratory-type ailments. We use eucalyptus herb in face steam for congestion or sinus difficulties and I create a light (and petroleum-free) version of Vapo-Rub for coughing and respiratory disease. The essential oil may be diluted with coconut oil or olive oil and be used topically on the feet and chest to assist unblock nasal pathways.

Ginger Capsules:
Ginger is wonderful for nausea, indigestion, stomach discomfort, and morning sickness. I also have some in the vehicle for motion sickness. It helps relieve the stomach after a digestive disease or food poisoning.

Echinacea:
I have a homemade echinacea tincture available for serious diseases. I don't use it

as a first choice, although it is beneficial in protracted sickness.

Peppermint Herb and Essential Oil:
Another powerful digestive herb. For an unsettled stomach or digestive ailment, the plant is put into tea. The tincture may be used internally or topically for headaches. When coupled with a few other digestive herbs, it creates a very efficient digestive aid and nausea treatment. We also use this essential oil in our handmade toothpaste.

Plantain:
You've undoubtedly plucked this as a weed without knowing it! I have the dried herb on hand at all times to put into a poultice for poison ivy, bites, stings, wounds, and infection. In a pinch, I've taken some off the ground, chewed it, and placed it on a bee sting for rapid pain relief.

Slippery Elm:

Helpful for painful or irritated throat or when you lose your voice. These lozenges taste excellent and are useful for youngsters with sore throats. The plant itself may be used in tinctures or teas for sore throat alleviation.

Apple Cider Vinegar:

I have a bottle of organic Apple Cider Vinegar with "the mother" on hand for digestive difficulties, indigestion, food poisoning, and more. Taken at a dosage of 1 teaspoon per 8 ounces of water every hour, it helps lessen the length of any form of sickness, however, it is tricky to convince youngsters to take it voluntarily.

Vitamin C– Helpful for all ailments, but notably flu-related illnesses. I keep the powder on hand since it is additive-free and can be put into meals or beverages to entice the kids to take it.

Aloe Vera Plant:

We have one growing in the home for burns and blisters.

Epsom Salt:

Good as a bath soak for weary muscles. Dissolved in water, it may also be a useful soak to help remove splinters.

Hydrogen Peroxide:

I have several bottles on hand at all times. It's wonderful for disinfecting, cleaning tiny wounds, and in my homemade OxyClean.

I also put a dropper full of hydrogen peroxide in the ear at the first symptom of an ear infection (but check with your doctor first) (but check with your doctor first). I let the peroxide in for 15 minutes or until it stops bubbling and then repeat on the other side.

Homemade Neosporin:

I create my own "boo-boo" lotion as my kids call it (no petroleum required) (no petroleum needed). I store it in little tins and lip chap containers for on-the-go size. I use this on scrapes, bruises, rashes, and everything else antibiotic ointment may be used on.

Witch Hazel:
I keep a gallon on hand for use on wounds, scratches, and cosmetic reasons. It creates a terrific skin toner and is helpful for the postpartum bottom.

Gelatin:
I consume gelatin frequently for its health advantages, but I also have it on hand for first aid and sickness. The natural gelatin in homemade chicken soup (from the bones and tissue) is one of the elements that makes it so nutritious during sickness. During any form of sickness, the sufferer obtains gelatin in numerous ways: in meals, homemade jello, smoothies, and hot tea.

Baking Soda:

Also a wonderful cure to have on hand. For severe heartburn or urinary tract infections, 1/4 tsp may be administered internally to assist ease fast. It may also be prepared into a poultice and used for spider bites.

Probiotics:
These are the probiotics we utilize throughout any disease and subsequently to heal gut flora. I've seen clients improve skin issues with frequent usage of probiotics, and I strongly prescribe them to expectant moms, since newborn newborns acquire their gut flora from their mothers. For youngsters who have frequent sickness and ear infections, probiotics may also tremendously assist.

Coconut Oil: - From skin salve to diaper cream, makeup remover, and even antifungal therapy, coconut oil is fantastic to keep around! I keep some in the natural first aid box to add treatments to take internally, use in tinctures, and apply topically to dry skin and chapped lips.

A Better-for-You Medicine Cabinet
The only true drugs you'll discover in my cupboard are from Genexa and their range of no dye, no preservative, additive-free medicines. They carry everything from pain relief to saline, as well as homeopathic remedies. You may also be able to get them at a local drugstore near you!

Other Natural First Aid Kit Supplies

Patch Bandages:
These bandages are constructed from 100% organic bamboo and are enhanced with coconut oil.
Butterfly Bandages/Gauze Superglue:– On small to severe skin cuts (not puncture wounds) use superglue and butterfly bandages. I've used this instead of stitches multiple times and it healed quickly and left

less scarring than the places I've had stitches.

This notably helps for the face and other prominent parts that scar readily or in the hair where conventional bandages might be difficult to apply. I've also put it on fingers or knuckles (I'm known for shredding knuckles when cooking) or other areas where band-aids won't stick nicely.

- Strips of sterilized muslin fabric in plastic bags for dressing wounds.
- Cut off wool sleeves from old sweaters to cover bandages and hold ice packs
- Hot water bottle
- Enema kit
- Bulb syringe and NoseFrida for assisting with congestion in youngsters
- Homemade ice pack (simply freeze liquid dish soap or rubbing alcohol in a double-bagged- ziplock bag and use as an ice pack.

Herbal treatments are something I always keep on hand for whatever life brings. They won't do me much good, however, if I can't locate what I need when I need it! Here's how to store and arrange your natural treatments, herbs, and more.

How to Store Your Natural Remedies

As my natural treatments began to surpass conventional ones, my collection expanded and increased. I'm pretty proud of my natural medicine cabinet, but it does take some maintenance. No one wants to discover a neglected, rotting ointment at the bottom of a pile.

By having my herbal medication organized, I can be sure to not only locate what I need but not squander what I have.

If you've ever heard of the KonMari approach (or even if you haven't), it may apply to organizing and storing natural remedies, too. It doesn't imply we have to store things in a certain method, but some of the underlying ideas are the same.

Declutter and get rid of unwanted natural treatments
Clean out and organize goods into groupings
Organize what's left
Unlike the traditional Marie Kondo technique, I'm not thanking my rotten salve before tossing it away, however. And my cough syrup may not inspire delight, but it's still helpful and required. First things first, let's talk about cleaning out our home remedies.

Gather it All Together
It's hard to arrange something you can't see or don't realize you have. I advise collecting together all of your nutritional supplements, herbs, essential oils, and natural cures in one spot, like the kitchen table. This way, you can quickly lay everything all out and

see what's there and how it will fit in the area.

Discard any things that are expired or no longer fresh. Here's a brief reference on the shelf life of many natural remedies:

Dried herbs: More delicate herbs, like chamomile blossoms, will survive for 1-2 years. Powdered herbs lose potency faster and last 6-12 months. Roots and bark (like echinacea root) can last longer, about 2-3 years. Just because a herb is older doesn't necessarily mean it's lost its potency. If the plant material has nice color and a pleasant aroma, it's still beneficial, albeit maybe not as powerful.

Fresh herbs: These will only stay approximately one week maximum in the fridge. Either utilize fresh medicinal herbs straight soon or dry them.

Glycerites: Tinctures prepared with glycerine, termed glycerites, will survive around one year.

Tinctures:
Alcohol tinctures with a high alcohol concentration will survive 2-5 years.
Essential oils: Citrus oils oxidize quickly and only persist for around 1-2 years. Thicker, base note oils often stay longer (up to 8 years) and may even enhance with age, including vetiver, patchouli, and myrrh. Here's a nice infographic from Plant Therapy with broad essential oil shelf life guidelines.

Salves and creams: It depends on the ingredients and if you used a preservative or something to slow oxidation (like vitamin E oil) (like vitamin E oil). Generally, DIY salves will last for six months to 3 years. If it's beginning to split or looks or smells wrong in any way, be safe and discard it.

Supplements, homeopathic medicines, and vitamins: Refer to the expiry date on the bottle since this changes.

Store water-based items in the fridge and utilize them within a week or so. This includes homemade lotion or after-sun spray. If you're using a natural antibacterial preservative, creams and lotions will remain a bit longer on the shelf.

Finding a Place to Store Your Natural Remedies

We want our remedies to be in a spot that's simple to get and makes sense for what we're utilizing them for. Essential oils for the bedroom diffuser might be placed on the dresser. I have magnesium oil and lotion bars on my bedside for when it's time to wind down at night.

Convenience is one thing, but we also have to consider storage conditions. Natural treatments aren't the same as FDA-approved prescription pharmaceuticals, and they need to be handled with great care. Herbs and essential oils should be kept in a cool, dark area, away from direct light and heat. The health advantages of these medicinal herbs fade if they're not preserved carefully.

Here are some areas where it is NOT advised to keep natural remedies:

Above or directly near appliances that let off heat and moisture, such as the stove, dishwasher, or refrigerator. That little cupboard over the stove is not the proper location for herbs!
In the bathroom or close to the shower. Bathrooms may become incredibly hot and heated and don't mix well with many natural cures.

Where tiny ones can reach them. While I'm not going to stress out if a toddler gets into the dried peppermint, some natural health things (like essential oils) need to be kept out of reach of inquisitive young hands.

With these limitations in mind, simply determine what makes sense for your family. Maybe that's a bookcase, a free-standing cabinet, or a kitchen cupboard (or 3!). Even if they're not all going to be housed in the same spot, choose spaces and containers that will accommodate the diverse goods in your home pharmacy.

Make Sure to Label Everything

Regular supplements and vitamins already come with labels, but homemade items are a different story. It's important to date and labels everything, so we know what it is. You may believe you'll remember that a sleep tincture was in that bottle, but as you acquire more things, you may rapidly become confused if herbal goods aren't labeled.

Write down the name of the herb and when you bought or gathered it.

List down the components and the date you produced the herbal treatment for salves, mixed tinctures, blended teas, etc.

Masking tape or address labels are also effective solutions. Masking tape is often simpler to remove if you wish to reuse and relabel the container for a future time.

I learned the importance of labeling everything to help stay organized (especially with kids!)

Time to Organize Your Natural Remedies
Once you've chosen a spot to keep your natural remedies and rejected what's harmful, it's time to start arranging. You may organize products by what you use the most, sort them alphabetically, or put all related items together (like all the dry herbs in one area) (like the dried herbs in one

spot). If specific family members have their items, you may organize things that way too.

Containers for Organizing Natural Remedies
There are several different possibilities, and it doesn't have to be pricey. It's usually ideal to keep herbs, essential oils, and tinctures in glass bottles for the greatest shelf life. Mason jars, weck jars, or even old glass food jars will work. If you prefer to keep dry herbs in the bags they came in, lay them upright in a row in a small container.

Tiered shelves are a fantastic use of space because you can see what's in the rear rows. Supplements, vitamins, tinctures, and essential oil bottles work nicely on tiered shelves.

Organizing containers, like these plastic bins, are wonderful for drawers.

Homeopathy bottles are lightweight and tend to tumble everywhere in my cupboard, so I prefer to confine them into their tiny bucket.

Be cautious to keep tincture bottles and essential oils in an upright posture so they don't leak. The rubber on the top of tincture dropper vials will start to disintegrate over time. A simple alternative is to remove the dropper top and replace it with a screw-top cap for tinctures that will be hanging about for a long.

Put things you use the most (such as daily vitamins) at the front or in the handiest areas. Items that I don't use often move to the rear. Something like this syrup for dry coughs is incredibly handy when I need it, but my kids don't have a sore throat every day. When I want to strengthen our immune systems throughout the winter months, I'll make sure our elderberry is handy to reach.

Chapter 5

Home treatments that are easy and efficient

Chances are you've tried a home remedy at some point: herbal drinks for cold, essential oils to dull a headache, plant-based vitamins for a better night's sleep. Maybe it was your granny or you heard about it online. The point is you tried it – and maybe now you're wondering, "Should I try it again?"

It's not apparent precisely what makes a home treatment perform the job. Is it a true physiological change in the body or more of a placebo effect? Thankfully, in recent decades, scientists have started exploring the same questions in a lab, and are discovering that some of our plant-based treatments aren't simply old wives' tales.

And therefore, for the skeptic who requires more than a placebo to feel healthy, we have your back. Here are the home cures supported by science:

Turmeric for pain and inflammation
Who hasn't heard of turmeric by now? Turmeric has been utilized, particularly in South Asia as a component of Ayurvedic treatment, for approximately 4,000 years. When it comes to established medical applications, the golden spice may be greatest for alleviating pain – especially pain connected with inflammation.

Several studies have indicated that curcumin is responsible for turmeric's "wow" impact. In one research, persons with arthritic paint rusted Sources noticed that their pain levels were decreased after taking 500 milligrams (mg) of curcumin than 50 mg of diclofenac sodium, an anti-inflammatory medicine.

Trusted Source backed up this pain treatment claim as well, adding that turmeric extract was as efficient as ibuprofen for alleviating pain.

Don't start crushing turmeric which stains significantly! for fast relief, however. The quantity of curcumin in turmeric is at most 3 percent, indicating you're better off taking curcumin pills for relief.

That's not to say a calming turmeric latte won't help. It's claimed that 2 to 5 grams (g) of the spice may still give some advantages. Just make sure you add black pepper to increase the absorption.

Drink a cup per day
Turmeric is about the long game. Consuming 1/2 to 1 1/2 tsp. of turmeric per day should start producing apparent advantages after four to eight weeks.

Chili peppers for pain and discomfort
This active component of chili peppers has a long history of usage in traditional medicine

and has steadily become increasingly acknowledged outside of homeopathy. Now, capsaicin is a common topical medication for controlling pain. It works by making an area of the skin feel heated, before gradually going numb.

Today, you can purchase a prescription capsaicin patch called Qutenza, which needs an extremely high dose of capsaicin — 8 percent trusted Source — to function.

So, when it comes to painful muscles or widespread body discomfort that won't leave you alone, and you have some hot peppers or cayenne pepper on hand? Make some capsaicin cream.

DIY capsaicin coconut oil cream
Mix 3 tbsp. of cayenne powder with 1 cup of coconut.
Heat the oil on low heat until it melts.
Stir the mixture vigorously for 5 minutes.

Remove from heat and pour into a basin. Let it firm up.

Massage into the skin when cold.

For an extra luxurious feel, whisk your coconut oil with a hand mixer so that it becomes light and fluffy.

It's vital to assess your response to the substance before taking it too intensively. You may also use jalapeño peppers, although the level of heat may vary depending on the pepper. Never use this cream over the face or eyes, and be sure to wear gloves while applying.

Ginger for pain and nausea
It's virtual law to try ginger when you have a cold, sore throat, or are suffering morning sickness and nausea. Making a cup is relatively standard: Grate it in your tea for a greater impact. But the second advantage of ginger that gets less acknowledged is its efficacy as an anti-inflammatory.

The next time you feel a bit sick and have a headache, try ginger. Ginger works differently than other pain medications that target inflammation. It prevents the production of specific kinds of inflammatory chemicals and breaks down existing inflammation via an antioxidant that interacts with acidity in the fluid between joints. Its anti-inflammatory effects are trusted sources that come without the dangers of nonsteroidal anti-inflammatory medications (NSAIDs) (NSAIDs).

Ginger tea recipe
Grate half an inch of raw ginger.
Boil 2 cups of water and pour over ginger.
Let sit for 5 to 10 minutes.
Add juice from a lemon, then add honey or agave nectar to taste.
Shiitake mushrooms for the long game
Lentinan, also known as AHCC or active hexose correlated compound, is an extract of shiitake mushrooms. It boosts antioxidant

and anti-inflammatory effects Trusted Source at a cellular level.

Trusted Source says that AHCC may aid with suppressing breast cancer cells, and its interaction with the immune system can help fight cancer

If you've found bone broth to be soothing, put in a few sliced shiitake mushrooms next time. One study trusted Source showed that consuming 5 to 10 g of shiitake mushrooms per day could increase human immune systems after four weeks.

Eucalyptus oil for pain alleviation
Eucalyptus oil comprises a component called 1,8-cineole, which may help reduce discomfort. The component produces a morphine-like effect when tested on mistrusted Sources.

And for the essential oils aficionados, you're in luck. Eucalyptus oil has been demonstrated to ease bodily aches even after inhalation. For aficionados of Vick's VapoRub, who have been breathing it as a home cure for congestion, well, eucalyptus oil is your magic ingredient.

However, breathing eucalyptus oil isn't for everyone. This oil may induce asthma and may be dangerous to dogs. It may also cause respiratory discomfort in babies.

Lavender for migraine and anxiety
Migraine attacks, headaches, anxiety, and overall emotions of (dis)stress? Inhaling lavender may assist with that. Studies indicate that lavender helps with:

migraine
decreasing anxiety or restlessness
memory issues while stressed and sleepTrusted Source
Drinking lavender tea or having a satchel for times of high stress is one approach to

alleviate anxiety and soothe the mind and body.

As an essential oil, it may also be blended with other plant oils for aromatherapy. One study trusted Source showed that in conjunction with sage and rose, lavender was beneficial in alleviating premenstrual syndrome (PMS) symptoms.

Caution
While lavender is a potent herb, it may come with unwanted effects. Directly applying essential oil without diluting it may irritate the skin or perhaps disrupt hormone levels. Always diffuse and dilute essential oils before using.

Mint for muscular pain and digestion

Mint, as basic as it seems, isn't straightforward. Depending on the kind, it might have varied applications and advantages.

For pain, you'll want to seek wintergreen, which possesses methyl salicylate, a chemical that may function similarly to capsaicin. Applying it might feel like a cold "burn" before the numbing effect takes in. This impact helps with joint and muscular discomfort.

The other mint kind that's widely utilized in traditional medicine is peppermint. A constituent in many various remedies, peppermint has been discovered to be very useful in helping relieve irritable bowel syndrome (IBS) symptoms.

Studies demonstrate that coupled with fiber, it helps lessen spasmsTrusted Source, as well as diarrhea and gastrointestinal paint rusted Source linked with IBS. Peppermint triggers an anti-pain channel in the colon, which lowers inflammatory discomfort in the digestive system. This most likely accounts for its success in treating IBS.

Beyond digestion and stomach difficulties, a peppermint oil pill or tea may also assist with headaches, colds, and other bodily discomforts.

Fenugreek for breastfeeding
Fenugreek seeds are commonly used in cooking throughout the Mediterranean and Asia, but this spice, which is related to cloves, has various medical properties.

When brewed into a tea, fenugreek may aid with milk production during breastfeedingTrusted Source. For persons having diarrhea, fenugreek is a wonderful water-soluble fiberTrusted Source to help firm up stools. If you're constipated, you certainly want to avoid these seeds.

As a supplement, fenugreek has also been discovered to decrease blood sugarTrusted Source, making it a popular help for those with diabetes. Fenugreek's significance here is due in part to its high fiber content, which may aid with boosting insulin functionTrusted Source.

Fenugreek in cooking
Fenugreek is typically crushed and used in curries, dry rubs, and teas. You may add it to your yogurt for a mild savory flavor, or sprinkle it over your salads.

Magnesium-rich meals for everything
Feeling muscular pains? Fatigue?
More migraine attacks? More inclined to slide into a dulled emotional state than usual? It could be a magnesium deficit. While magnesium is generally spoken about in terms of the formation and preservation of bones, it's also crucial in nerve and muscle function.

But studies reveal that approximately half of the U.S. population doesn't obtain their needed quantity of magnesiumTrusted Source. So, if you've ever complained of these symptoms and received a little curt "eat spinach" comment in return, know that it's not wholly baseless.

Spinach, almonds, avocados, and even dark chocolate are all high in magnesium. You don't need a supplement to cure magnesium insufficiency.

When it comes to mood, magnesium may also aid. Magnesium interacts with the parasympathetic nervous system, which keeps you calm and relaxed, indicating that eating a magnesium-rich diet can assist with stress alleviation. Trusted Source

Foods rich in magnesium
lentils, beans, chickpeas, and peas
tofu
Whole grains
fatty fish, including salmon, mackerel, and halibut
bananas

Make careful you apply home treatments appropriately

Certain people may also be more sensitive to dosage amounts, so if you're on any medication or live with a condition that's affected by your diet, talk to a doctor before consuming these foods regularly. And if you have an allergic reaction or worsening symptoms from any home remedy, speak to a doctor right away.

Keep in mind that home treatments may not always be safe and helpful for you. While they are validated by scientific research, a single study or clinical trial doesn't necessarily encompass various populations or bodies. What research indicates as useful may not always work for you.

Many of the cures we mentioned above are ones we grew up with, ones that families have handed down and brought us up on since we were young, and we look forward to leaning back on them when we need comfort.

Printed in Great Britain
by Amazon

27138613R00066